Wellness Health Easy to Use Guide for Beginners

Understanding the Importance of Wellness Health

By

Raibeart Scott

Copyright@2023

Table of Contents

CHAPTER 1

Introduction

1.1 Welcome to the Wellness Health Guide

Welcome to the "Wellness Health Guide," a comprehensive resource designed to empower beginners on their journey towards improved well-being and a healthier lifestyle. In a world inundated with information on health and wellness, embarking on this path can often feel overwhelming. This guide aims to demystify the process, making it accessible and easy to understand for individuals of all backgrounds and ages.

In our fast-paced lives, it's easy to neglect our health. The daily demands of work, family, and personal commitments often lead us to put our well-being on the backburner. However, the consequences of neglecting our health can be far-reaching, affecting not only our physical health but also our mental and emotional well-being.

This guide is here to remind you that your health should be a top priority, and it doesn't have to be an intimidating or complex endeavor. Whether you're just starting your wellness journey or looking for ways to refine your existing habits, you'll find valuable insights, practical tips, and actionable advice within these pages.

1.2 Why Wellness Health Matters

Wellness health matters for a multitude of reasons that extend far beyond the absence of illness. It encompasses a holistic approach to health, focusing on not only the physical aspect but also the mental, emotional, and social dimensions of well-being. Here are some compelling reasons why wellness health should be a fundamental part of your life:

1. Improved Quality of Life: When you prioritize your wellness health, you can expect to enjoy a better quality of life. This includes increased energy levels, enhanced mental clarity, better mood, and a greater sense of overall vitality. You'll be better equipped to tackle life's challenges and enjoy its pleasures.

2. Prevention and Longevity: Investing in wellness health is like investing in your future. By adopting healthy habits and making smart choices, you reduce the risk of chronic diseases such as heart disease, diabetes, and obesity. It's not just about adding years to your life but adding life to your years.

3. Mental and Emotional Well-being: Wellness health isn't just about physical fitness; it also includes mental and emotional well-being. When you nurture your mental health, you can better manage stress, anxiety, and depression, leading to greater resilience and emotional balance.

4. Stronger Relationships: Good health can positively impact your relationships. When you feel your best, you're more likely to engage with others in a positive and meaningful way. Healthy habits can also inspire those around you to make positive changes in their lives.

5. Productivity and Fulfillment: Wellness health can boost your productivity and overall life satisfaction. When your body and mind are functioning optimally, you can excel in your personal and professional endeavors, leading to a more fulfilling and successful life.

6. Reducing Healthcare Costs: Preventative measures are often more cost-effective than treating illness. By focusing on wellness health, you may reduce your healthcare expenses in the long run, freeing up resources for other aspects of your life.

7. Empowerment and Self-Care:
Prioritizing wellness health is an act
of self-care and empowerment. It's a
way to take control of your life and
make choices that align with your
values and goals. It's a declaration that
you are worth the effort it takes to live
a healthier and happier life.

In essence, wellness health is the
foundation upon which a fulfilling
and vibrant life is built. It's about
nurturing yourself on all levels—
physically, mentally, emotionally, and
socially. This guide will walk you
through the steps to help you embrace
wellness health, providing you with
the tools and knowledge you need to
embark on this transformative
journey. So, let's get started on the
path to a healthier, happier you.

CHAPTER 2

Understanding Wellness Health

2.1 What Is Wellness Health

Wellness health, often simply referred to as "wellness," is a multifaceted and holistic approach to health and well-being. It goes beyond the absence of disease and encompasses various dimensions that contribute to a person's overall quality of life. At its core, wellness health is about achieving a state of optimal physical, mental, emotional, and social well-being.

Here are some key aspects that define wellness health:

- **Physical Health:** This dimension relates to the state of your physical body. It includes factors such as nutrition, exercise, sleep, and disease prevention. Physical health aims to ensure your body functions optimally and remains free from illness to the extent possible.

- **Mental Health:** Mental wellness pertains to your cognitive and emotional well-being. It encompasses factors like stress management, resilience, positive thinking, and emotional balance. Mental health is essential for maintaining a clear mind and healthy emotional responses to life's challenges.

- **Emotional Health:** Emotional wellness focuses on understanding and managing your emotions effectively. It involves recognizing and expressing your feelings in a healthy way and nurturing positive emotional experiences. Emotional health is vital for building strong relationships and coping with life's ups and downs.

- **Social Health:** Social wellness involves your interactions and relationships with others. It encompasses aspects such as communication skills, social support, and maintaining healthy connections with friends, family, and the community. A strong social network is a cornerstone of well-being.

- **Environmental Health:** Environmental wellness emphasizes the importance of the physical spaces in which you live and work. It includes factors like air and water quality, safety, and sustainability. Being in a clean and safe environment can positively impact your overall wellness.

- **Occupational Health:** Occupational wellness relates to your job or career satisfaction and work-life balance. It involves finding purpose and fulfillment in your work, managing stress related to your job, and maintaining a healthy balance between work and personal life.

- **Spiritual Health:** Spiritual wellness doesn't necessarily refer to religious beliefs but rather to finding meaning and purpose in life. It involves connecting with your values, beliefs, and a sense of purpose that transcends day-to-day existence.

- **Intellectual Health:** Intellectual wellness involves keeping your mind engaged and active. It includes pursuing knowledge, critical thinking, problem-solving, and continuous learning. Intellectual stimulation

contributes to a sense of
fulfillment and growth.

- **Financial Health:** Financial wellness focuses on managing your finances in a way that supports your overall well-being. It includes budgeting, saving, investing, and making informed financial decisions to achieve your goals and reduce stress related to money.

- **Cultural Health:** Cultural wellness recognizes the importance of respecting and embracing cultural diversity. It involves understanding and appreciating different cultures, customs, and traditions, which can lead to greater tolerance and inclusivity.

Understanding wellness health means recognizing that all these dimensions are interconnected. Neglecting one aspect can impact the others, so a holistic approach to well-being involves addressing and nurturing each dimension.

2.2 The Benefits of Prioritizing Wellness Health

Prioritizing wellness health offers a multitude of benefits that can positively impact every aspect of your life:

- **Enhanced Quality of Life:** Wellness health leads to a higher quality of life characterized by better physical health, emotional well-being, and a stronger sense of purpose.

- **Disease Prevention:** A focus on wellness can reduce the risk of chronic diseases and health issues, ultimately leading to a longer and healthier life.

- **Improved Mental Resilience:** Mental wellness practices help you cope with stress, anxiety, and adversity more effectively.

- **Stronger Relationships:** Social and emotional wellness fosters healthier connections with others, leading to more fulfilling relationships.

- **Increased Productivity:** When you feel your best, you're more productive and better able to achieve your personal and professional goals.

- **Greater Satisfaction:**
Wellness health can lead to
increased life satisfaction as
you align your actions with
your values and pursue a
balanced life.

CHAPTER 3

Getting Started

Embarking on your wellness journey is an exciting and empowering endeavor. To ensure a successful and sustainable path toward improved well-being, it's essential to begin with a solid foundation.

3.1 Setting Your Wellness Goals

Before you can make meaningful progress, it's crucial to define your wellness goals. These goals will serve as your roadmap and motivation throughout your journey. Here's how to set effective wellness goals:

- **Be Specific:** Clearly define what you want to achieve. Instead of a vague goal like "get healthier," specify what that means to you. For example, "lose 10 pounds in three months" or "reduce stress through meditation."

- **Make Them Measurable:** Ensure your goals are quantifiable so that you can track your progress. Use concrete metrics, such as weight, exercise duration, or weekly meditation sessions.

- **Set Achievable Goals:** While it's essential to aim high, make sure your goals are realistic and attainable. Setting overly ambitious goals can lead to frustration and burnout.

- **Relevance:** Align your goals with your values and priorities. Ask yourself why these goals matter to you and how achieving them will improve your life.

- **Time-Bound:** Set a timeframe for achieving your goals. This adds a sense of urgency and helps you stay accountable. For instance, "lose 10 pounds in three months" sets a clear deadline.

- **Break Them Down:** If your goals are substantial, break them into smaller, manageable steps. This makes the journey less daunting and allows you to celebrate smaller victories along the way.

- **Write Them Down:** Put your goals in writing. This reinforces your commitment and makes them more tangible.

wellness goals are highly individual. Your goals should reflect what you genuinely want to achieve and the areas of your well-being that are most important to you. Whether it's weight loss, improved fitness, stress reduction, or enhanced mental clarity, setting clear and personalized goals is the first step toward success.

3.2 Assessing Your Current Health

To create an effective wellness plan, you need to have a clear understanding of your current health status. This assessment provides you with valuable baseline information and helps identify areas that need attention. Here's how to assess your current health:

- **Medical Check-Up:** Schedule a comprehensive medical check-up with your healthcare provider. This includes measurements of vital signs like blood pressure, cholesterol levels, and body mass index (BMI). Discuss any existing health conditions or concerns.

- **Health History:** Reflect on your medical history and any family history of illnesses. This can help identify genetic factors that may influence your wellness journey.

- **Physical Fitness:** Assess your current physical fitness level. You can perform simple tests like measuring your flexibility, endurance, and strength. Note any physical limitations or discomfort you experience during exercise.

- **Dietary Habits:** Keep a food diary for a week to track your eating habits. Note what you eat, portion sizes, and meal timings. This will give you insights into your nutritional choices.

- **Mental and Emotional Well-being:** Reflect on your mental and emotional state. Are you experiencing high levels of stress, anxiety, or mood swings? Recognizing these challenges is the first step in addressing them.

- **Sleep Patterns:** Evaluate your sleep patterns. Are you getting enough restful sleep, or do you struggle with insomnia or disrupted sleep? Sleep is a critical component of wellness health.

- **Lifestyle Habits:** Assess your lifestyle habits, including smoking, alcohol consumption, and recreational drug use. Identify areas where changes may be necessary for better health.

3.3 Creating a Wellness Plan

With a clear understanding of your wellness goals and your current health status, you're now ready to create a personalized wellness plan. A wellness plan is a comprehensive strategy that outlines the actions and steps you'll take to achieve your goals. Here's how to create an effective plan:

- **Prioritize Your Goals:** Start by prioritizing your wellness goals. Determine which goals are most important to you and which ones you want to tackle first.

- **Break Goals into Action Steps:** Divide each goal into smaller, actionable steps. These steps should be specific and achievable.

- **Create a Schedule:** Establish a realistic schedule for implementing each action step. Determine how often you'll perform these steps and when you'll start.

- **Gather Resources:** Identify the resources you'll need to support your wellness plan. This may include exercise equipment, healthy recipes, meditation apps, or support from healthcare professionals.

- **Accountability:** Share your wellness plan with a trusted friend or family member who can hold you accountable. You can also consider working with a wellness coach or personal trainer.

- **Track Progress:** Set up a system for tracking your progress. This could be a journal, a mobile app, or a spreadsheet. Regularly review your progress and make adjustments as needed.

- **Celebrate Achievements:** Celebrate your successes, no matter how small they may seem. Recognizing your accomplishments reinforces your commitment to your wellness journey.

Your wellness plan is a flexible tool. It should adapt to your changing needs and circumstances. As you progress on your journey, you may need to revise and refine your plan to stay aligned with your goals.

CHAPTER 4

Nutrition for Beginners

Nutrition plays a fundamental role in your overall health and well-being. It's a cornerstone of wellness health, and understanding the basics of balanced nutrition is essential for beginners on their wellness journey.

4.1 Basics of Balanced Nutrition

Balanced nutrition involves consuming a variety of foods that provide your body with the necessary nutrients in the right proportions. Here are the key components of balanced nutrition:

- **Macronutrients:** These are the nutrients your body needs in large quantities:

  - **Carbohydrates:** They are the primary source of energy. Choose complex carbohydrates like whole grains, fruits, vegetables, and legumes over simple sugars.

  - **Proteins:** Essential for building and repairing

tissues. Include lean sources of protein like poultry, fish, beans, and tofu.

- **Fats:** Provide energy and support various bodily functions. Opt for healthy fats such as those found in avocados, nuts, seeds, and olive oil.

- **Micronutrients:** These are essential vitamins and minerals that your body requires in smaller quantities:

  - **Vitamins:** Include a variety of fruits and vegetables in your diet to get a wide range of vitamins, such as vitamin C, vitamin A, and vitamin D.

- **Minerals:** Consume foods rich in minerals like calcium (found in dairy products), iron (in lean meats and beans), and potassium (in bananas and spinach).

- **Fiber:** Dietary fiber is crucial for digestive health and helps maintain stable blood sugar levels. It's abundant in fruits, vegetables, whole grains, and legumes.

- **Hydration:** Proper hydration is vital for overall health. Drink plenty of water throughout the day, and limit sugary beverages.

- **Portion Control:** Pay attention to portion sizes to avoid overeating. Use smaller plates and practice mindful eating to better gauge your hunger and fullness cues.

- **Moderation:** Enjoy all foods in moderation. Avoid extreme diets or strict food restrictions, as they can be challenging to maintain and may lead to nutrient deficiencies.

- **Balanced Meals:** Aim for balanced meals that include a source of protein, carbohydrates, and healthy fats. Include a variety of colorful fruits and vegetables to ensure you're getting a range of nutrients.

- **Limit Processed Foods:** Minimize the consumption of highly processed and sugary foods, which can contribute to health problems.

- **Read Labels:** When purchasing packaged foods, read nutrition labels to make informed choices. Pay attention to ingredients, serving sizes, and added sugars.

4.2 Meal Planning Tips

Meal planning is a valuable tool for maintaining a balanced diet. It helps you make healthier food choices, save time and money, and reduce food waste. Here are some meal planning tips for beginners:

- **Set Realistic Goals:** Start with achievable meal planning goals. For instance, plan meals for a few days or a week at a time before attempting more extended planning.

- **Create a Weekly Menu:** Plan your meals for the upcoming week. Include breakfast, lunch, dinner, and snacks. Consider your schedule and choose recipes that suit your lifestyle.

- **Use a Planner or App:** A meal planning app or a simple pen-and-paper planner can help you organize your meals and grocery lists.

- **Choose Nutrient-Rich Foods:** Base your meals around whole foods like lean proteins, whole grains, and plenty of fruits and vegetables.

- **Prep in Advance:** Spend some time prepping ingredients in advance, such as chopping vegetables or marinating proteins. This can save you time during busy weekdays.

- **Batch Cooking:** Cook in larger quantities and freeze extra portions for future meals. This is especially helpful for busy days when you don't have time to cook from scratch.

- **Mix and Match:** Create versatile components that you can mix and match to create different meals. For example, cook a batch of quinoa, roast a variety of vegetables, and prepare different proteins to combine in various ways throughout the week.

- **Grocery Shopping:** Make a shopping list based on your meal plan to avoid impulse purchases and ensure you have all the ingredients you need.

- **Stay Flexible:** Life can be unpredictable. Be prepared to adjust your meal plan if needed but aim to make healthier choices even when dining out or ordering takeout.

- **Plan for Snacks:** Include healthy snacks in your meal plan to curb mid-day cravings. Options like yogurt, nuts, or cut-up vegetables with hummus can satisfy hunger between meals.

- **Track Your Progress:** Keep a record of your meals, including what worked well and what you'd like to improve. Adjust your meal planning approach based on your experiences.

Meal planning is a skill that develops over time. Be patient with yourself and make adjustments as you learn more about your preferences and nutritional needs. With practice, meal planning can become a valuable tool in your journey toward balanced nutrition and overall wellness.

4.3 Nutrient-Rich Foods to Include

Including nutrient-rich foods in your diet is a key aspect of balanced nutrition. These foods provide essential vitamins, minerals, fiber, and other beneficial compounds that support your overall health and well-being. Here are some nutrient-rich foods to consider including in your meals:

1. Fruits: Fruits are rich in vitamins, antioxidants, and dietary fiber. Opt for a variety of fruits like berries, citrus fruits, apples, and bananas.

2. Vegetables: Vegetables provide a wide range of vitamins, minerals, and antioxidants. Leafy greens, broccoli, carrots, peppers, and sweet potatoes are excellent choices.

3. Whole Grains: Whole grains are a source of complex carbohydrates, fiber, and essential nutrients. Choose options like brown rice, quinoa, oats, whole wheat pasta, and whole grain bread.

4. Lean Proteins: Lean protein sources are essential for muscle health and overall well-being. Include skinless poultry, lean cuts of beef or pork, fish, tofu, beans, and lentils.

5. Dairy or Dairy Alternatives: Dairy products like low-fat yogurt and milk are rich in calcium and protein.

If you're lactose intolerant or prefer non-dairy options, choose fortified plant-based milks like almond, soy, or oat milk.

6. Nuts and Seeds: These are excellent sources of healthy fats, protein, and various vitamins and minerals. Almonds, walnuts, chia seeds, and flaxseeds are great choices.

7. Healthy Fats: Include sources of healthy fats like avocados, olive oil, and fatty fish (e.g., salmon and trout). These fats support heart health and brain function.

8. Beans and Legumes: Beans and legumes are rich in fiber, protein, and various nutrients. Options include black beans, chickpeas, lentils, and kidney beans.

9. Eggs: Eggs are a versatile source of protein and essential nutrients like choline. They can be prepared in various ways, from boiled to scrambled.

10. Berries: Berries such as blueberries, strawberries, and raspberries are packed with antioxidants and vitamins while being relatively low in calories.

11. Dark Leafy Greens: Foods like spinach, kale, and Swiss chard are nutrient powerhouses, providing vitamins, minerals, and antioxidants.

12. Seafood: Fatty fish like salmon, mackerel, and sardines are rich in omega-3 fatty acids, which support heart and brain health.

13. Colorful Vegetables: Aim to eat a variety of colorful vegetables as different colors often signify different nutrients. For example, red and orange vegetables are high in vitamin C and beta-carotene.

14. Herbs and Spices: Many herbs and spices have health benefits. Include garlic, turmeric, ginger, and cinnamon in your cooking for added flavor and potential health advantages.

15. Water: Staying hydrated is crucial for overall health. Water helps with digestion, temperature regulation, and nutrient absorption. Drink water throughout the day to maintain proper hydration.

4.4 Avoiding Common Nutrition Mistakes

While focusing on nutrient-rich foods is important, it's also crucial to avoid common nutrition mistakes that can hinder your wellness journey. Here are some pitfalls to watch out for:

1. Excessive Sugar: Limit the intake of added sugars found in sugary beverages, candies, and processed foods. Excessive sugar consumption can contribute to weight gain and health issues.

2. Processed Foods: Minimize the consumption of highly processed foods like chips, fast food, and sugary cereals. They are often high in unhealthy fats, sodium, and additives.

3. Skipping Meals: Skipping meals can lead to overeating later in the day and fluctuations in blood sugar levels. Aim for regular, balanced meals and snacks.

4. Fad Diets: Avoid extreme diets that promise quick results. They are often unsustainable and may lack essential nutrients.

5. Ignoring Portion Sizes: Be mindful of portion sizes to avoid overeating. Use smaller plates and listen to your body's hunger and fullness cues.

6. Not Reading Labels: Pay attention to food labels to understand what you're eating. Look for hidden sugars, unhealthy fats, and additives.

7. Not Drinking Enough Water: Dehydration can lead to fatigue and confusion. Ensure you drink enough water throughout the day.

8. Skipping Breakfast: Breakfast provides essential energy for the day. Skipping it can lead to poor concentration and overeating later on.

9. Emotional Eating: Avoid using food as a coping mechanism for stress or emotions. Seek healthier ways to manage your emotions, such as exercise or mindfulness.

10. Lack of Variety: Eating the same foods regularly may lead to nutrient deficiencies. Aim for a diverse diet to ensure you get a wide range of nutrients.

11. Ignoring Dietary Restrictions: If you have dietary restrictions or food allergies, it's essential to plan meals carefully and seek suitable alternatives to ensure balanced nutrition.

Incorporating nutrient-rich foods while avoiding common nutrition mistakes can help you maintain a balanced and healthy diet. Remember that it's okay to indulge occasionally, but the foundation of your diet should consist of foods that nourish and support your overall well-being.

CHAPTER 5

Exercise and Fitness

Exercise and physical activity are integral components of wellness health. Regular exercise not only benefits your physical health but also contributes to mental and emotional well-being.

5.1 Starting an Exercise Routine

Starting an exercise routine can be both exciting and challenging. Here's a step-by-step guide to help you begin:

Assess Your Current Fitness Level: Begin by assessing your current fitness level. This includes evaluating your cardiovascular endurance, strength, flexibility, and any physical limitations. You can use fitness assessment tools or consult with a fitness professional if needed.

Set Clear Goals: Define your fitness goals. Whether it's weight loss, increased strength, improved flexibility, or overall fitness, having clear objectives will keep you motivated and focused.

Choose Activities You Enjoy: Select physical activities that you enjoy. Whether it's dancing, swimming, cycling, or hiking, engaging in activities you find enjoyable increases the likelihood that you'll stick with your routine.

Start Slowly: If you're new to exercise or haven't been active for a while, start slowly. Begin with shorter workouts at a lower intensity and gradually increase the duration and intensity over time.

Create a Schedule: Establish a regular exercise schedule that fits into your daily routine. Consistency is key to long-term success.

Warm-Up and Cool Down: Always include warm-up and cool-down exercises in your routine. This helps prevent injuries and aids in muscle recovery.

Listen to Your Body: Pay attention to your body's signals. If you experience pain, dizziness, or extreme fatigue during exercise, stop and seek guidance from a healthcare professional.

Stay Hydrated: Drink water before, during, and after your workouts to stay properly hydrated.

Seek Professional Guidance: If you're unsure about how to start or need personalized guidance, consider working with a certified personal trainer or fitness coach.

5.2 Types of Physical Activities

There are various types of physical activities to choose from, depending on your preferences and fitness goals. Here are some options to consider:

Cardiovascular Activities:

- **Walking:** A low-impact exercise that's accessible to most people.

- **Running:** Provides a great cardiovascular workout and can be adapted to various fitness levels.

- **Cycling:** Whether on a stationary bike or outdoors, cycling is an excellent way to improve cardiovascular fitness.

- **Swimming:** A full-body workout that's easy on the joints.

- **Dancing:** Fun and rhythmic, dancing can be a great way to stay active.

Strength Training:

- **Weight Lifting:** Using free weights or resistance machines to build muscle strength.

- **Bodyweight Exercises:** Exercises like push-ups, squats, and planks require no equipment and can be done anywhere.

- **Resistance Bands:** These portable bands offer resistance for strength training exercises.

- **Yoga:** Combines strength, flexibility, and balance, and can also promote relaxation.

Flexibility and Balance:

- **Stretching:** Incorporate stretching exercises to improve flexibility and reduce the risk of injury.

- **Pilates:** Focuses on core strength, flexibility, and balance.

- **Tai Chi:** An ancient practice that promotes balance, flexibility, and relaxation.

Sports and Recreation:

- **Tennis, basketball, or soccer:** Team sports offer both physical activity and social interaction.

- **Hiking:** A great way to connect with nature while getting a workout.

- **Golf:** While it can be leisurely, walking the course and swinging the clubs provide exercise.

5.3 Building Strength and Endurance

Building strength and endurance is essential for overall fitness. Here are some strategies to help you in this regard:

Progressive Overload: Gradually increase the intensity of your workouts by adding weight, increasing reps or sets, or adjusting the difficulty of exercises. This progressive approach challenges your muscles and helps you build strength and endurance over time.

Balanced Routine: Include a mix of cardiovascular, strength, and flexibility exercises in your routine. This ensures that you work different muscle groups and maintain overall fitness.

Consistency: Stick to your exercise schedule consistently. Consistency is crucial for seeing progress in strength and endurance.

Rest and Recovery: Allow your muscles time to recover between intense workouts. Overtraining can lead to injuries and hinder progress. Ensure you get adequate sleep and practice recovery techniques like stretching and foam rolling.

Proper Form: Focus on maintaining proper form during exercises to prevent injuries and maximize effectiveness.

Nutrition: A balanced diet that supports your energy needs and muscle recovery is essential for building strength and endurance. Consult with a nutritionist if needed.

5.4 Staying Motivated

Staying motivated to exercise can be challenging, but there are strategies to help you stay on track:

Set Realistic Goals: Set achievable fitness goals and track your progress. Celebrate your accomplishments along the way.

Find Accountability: Exercise with a friend or join a fitness class to stay accountable. Sharing your goals with someone else can be motivating.

Variety: Keep your workouts interesting by trying new activities or varying your routine. This prevents boredom and plateaus.

Reward Yourself: Treat yourself to rewards when you reach fitness milestones. It can be as simple as buying new workout gear or enjoying a healthy treat.

Mindfulness: Practice mindfulness during your workouts. Pay attention to how exercise makes you feel, both physically and mentally.

Visualize Success: Visualize yourself achieving your fitness goals. Visualization can boost motivation and confidence.

Plan Ahead: Schedule your workouts in advance, so they become a non-negotiable part of your day.

Track Your Progress: Keep a fitness journal or use apps to track your workouts and see how far you've come.

Stay Informed: Continuously educate yourself about exercise and nutrition. Learning about the benefits of physical activity can boost motivation.

Exercise is a long-term commitment to your well-being. It's normal to have days when motivation wanes, but by implementing these strategies, you can stay motivated and continue reaping the physical and mental benefits of regular physical activity.

CHAPTER 6

Mental Well-being

Mental well-being is a vital aspect of overall health and wellness. It encompasses your emotional, psychological, and social well-being, influencing how you think, feel, and act.

6.1 The Importance of Mental Health

Mental health is as important as physical health, and the two are closely interconnected. Here's why mental health is crucial:

Emotional Well-being: Good mental health allows you to manage your emotions effectively, fostering positive experiences and healthy relationships.

Cognitive Function: Mental health influences your cognitive abilities, including memory, problem-solving, and decision-making.

Stress Management: It equips you with the resilience and coping strategies to deal with life's challenges and stressors.

Physical Health: Mental health affects physical health outcomes, including the immune system, cardiovascular health, and overall longevity.

Quality of Life: Mental health plays a significant role in your overall quality of life, contributing to happiness and life satisfaction.

Social Connections: It influences your ability to form and maintain social connections and enjoy meaningful relationships.

Productivity: Good mental health enhances productivity, creativity, and performance in various aspects of life.

6.2 Stress Management Techniques

Stress is a common part of life, but chronic stress can have detrimental effects on mental health. Learning effective stress management techniques can help maintain mental well-being:

1. Mindfulness Meditation: Practice mindfulness to stay present and reduce stress. Mindful breathing and meditation exercises can be helpful.

2. Exercise: Regular physical activity releases endorphins, which are natural mood lifters. Exercise is an effective stress reducer.

3. Relaxation Techniques: Try relaxation methods like deep breathing, progressive muscle relaxation, or yoga to alleviate stress.

4. Time Management: Organize your time effectively to reduce the feeling of being overwhelmed. Prioritize tasks and break them into manageable steps.

5. Healthy Lifestyle: Maintain a balanced diet, get adequate sleep, and limit caffeine and alcohol intake to support stress resilience.

6. Seek Support: Talk to friends, family, or a therapist when you're feeling stressed. Sharing your feelings can provide relief and perspective.

7. Problem-Solving: Break down stressful situations into smaller problems and work on solutions. Problem-solving can help reduce stressors.

8. Set Boundaries: Establish healthy boundaries in your personal and professional life to prevent excessive stress.

9. Journaling: Keeping a journal allows you to express your thoughts and feelings, helping you gain insight and manage stress.

10. Hobbies and Leisure: Engage in activities you enjoy to unwind and relax. Hobbies and leisure pursuits can be effective stress relievers.

6.3 Cultivating a Positive Mindset

A positive mindset can enhance mental well-being and resilience. Here's how to cultivate one:

Practice Gratitude: Regularly express gratitude for the positive aspects of your life. This can improve overall happiness and outlook.

Challenge Negative Thoughts: Be mindful of negative self-talk and challenge it with positive and realistic affirmations.

Self-Compassion: Treat yourself with kindness and understanding. Avoid harsh self-criticism.

Foster Optimism: Focus on the positive aspects of situations and cultivate a hopeful attitude toward the future.

Embrace Failure as Learning: View failures as opportunities for growth and learning rather than as setbacks.

Surround Yourself with Positivity: Spend time with positive and supportive people who uplift your spirits.

Engage in Positive Activities:
Participate in activities that bring joy
and satisfaction. Positive experiences
contribute to a positive mindset.

Mindful Living: Practice
mindfulness to stay present and
nonjudgmental. This can help you
appreciate the small pleasures in life.

6.4 Seeking Professional Help When Needed

It's essential to recognize when you
may need professional assistance for
your mental well-being:

Persistent Symptoms: If you
experience persistent symptoms of
depression, anxiety, or other mental
health conditions, seek help. These
symptoms may include intense

sadness, panic attacks, or intrusive thoughts.

Functional Impairment: When mental health issues significantly impact your daily functioning, such as work, relationships, or self-care, professional support is crucial.

Suicidal Thoughts: If you have thoughts of self-harm or suicide, it's an emergency. Reach out to a mental health crisis hotline or seek immediate help from a healthcare professional.

Lack of Coping Strategies: If you find it challenging to cope with stress, emotions, or life's challenges, a therapist can provide valuable tools and guidance.

Quality of Life: If your mental health is affecting your overall quality of life and well-being, consider therapy or counseling to address the underlying issues.

Supportive Professionals: Mental health professionals, including psychologists, psychiatrists, counselors, and therapists, can offer tailored treatment and support. They can provide therapy, medication, or a combination of both.

Stigma: Remember that seeking help for mental health is a sign of strength, not weakness. Stigma should not deter you from getting the support you need.

Prioritizing mental health is a fundamental aspect of overall well-being. By understanding its importance, practicing stress management techniques, cultivating a positive mindset, and seeking professional help when necessary, you can enhance your mental well-being and lead a healthier and more fulfilling life.

CHAPTER 7

Sleep and Rest

Sleep and rest are essential components of well-being that often get overlooked in our busy lives.

7.1 The Role of Sleep in Wellness

Understanding the importance of sleep-in wellness is critical for overall health and quality of life. Sleep plays several vital roles:

Physical Restoration: During deep sleep stages, the body repairs and regenerates tissues, supports muscle growth, and strengthens the immune system.

Mental Rejuvenation: Sleep is crucial for cognitive functions like memory consolidation, problem-solving, and learning. It also helps regulate mood and emotions.

Energy and Alertness: Adequate sleep ensures you wake up feeling refreshed and energized, ready to face the day with focus and alertness.

Metabolic Health: Sleep influences hormones that regulate appetite and metabolism. Poor sleep can lead to weight gain and an increased risk of metabolic conditions like diabetes.

Emotional Well-being: Quality sleep is linked to emotional stability and better stress management.

Cardiovascular Health: Chronic sleep deprivation has been associated with an increased risk of heart disease, hypertension, and stroke.

7.2 Establishing Healthy Sleep Habits

To improve your sleep and overall wellness, consider these healthy sleep habits:

Stick to a Sleep Schedule: Go to bed and wake up at the same time every day, even on weekends. This helps regulate your body's internal clock.

Create a Relaxing Bedtime Routine: Establish calming pre-sleep rituals, such as reading, gentle stretching, or taking a warm bath, to signal to your body that it's time to wind down.

Optimize Your Sleep Environment: Make your bedroom conducive to sleep by keeping it dark, quiet, and cool. Invest in a comfortable mattress and pillows.

Limit Screen Time: Reduce exposure to screens (phones, tablets, TVs) before bedtime, as the blue light emitted can interfere with the production of melatonin, a sleep-inducing hormone.

Watch Your Diet: Avoid heavy meals, caffeine, and alcohol close to bedtime. These substances can disrupt sleep.

Exercise Regularly: Engage in regular physical activity, but avoid strenuous exercise too close to bedtime, as it may be stimulating.

Limit Naps: If you need to nap during the day, keep it short (20-30 minutes) and early in the afternoon to avoid interfering with nighttime sleep.

Manage Stress: Practice relaxation techniques like meditation, deep breathing, or progressive muscle relaxation to manage stress, which can disrupt sleep.

Monitor Your Sleep: Keep a sleep journal to track your sleep patterns and identify any recurring issues.

Limit Bedtime Clock Watching: Constantly checking the time when you can't sleep can create anxiety and make it even harder to fall asleep.

Limit Exposure to Bright Light in the Evening: Exposure to natural or artificial bright light in the evening can disrupt your circadian rhythm. Consider dimming lights in the hours leading up to bedtime.

7.3 Dealing with Sleep Disorders

If you consistently have trouble sleeping despite practicing good sleep hygiene, you may have a sleep disorder. Common sleep disorders include:

Insomnia: Characterized by difficulty falling asleep, staying asleep, or waking up too early. It can result from stress, anxiety, or other underlying factors.

Sleep Apnea: A condition in which breathing repeatedly stops and starts during sleep. It often leads to snoring and excessive daytime sleepiness.

Restless Legs Syndrome (RLS): An uncomfortable sensation in the legs that leads to an irresistible urge to move them, often disrupting sleep.

Narcolepsy: A neurological disorder that causes excessive daytime sleepiness and sudden, uncontrollable sleep attacks.

Parasomnias: These include sleepwalking, night terrors, and REM sleep behavior disorder, where individuals physically act out their dreams during sleep.

If you suspect you have a sleep disorder, it's essential to consult a healthcare professional or sleep specialist. They can diagnose the condition and recommend appropriate treatment, which may include lifestyle changes, therapy, medication, or devices like continuous positive airway pressure (CPAP) machines for sleep apnea.

Prioritizing sleep and adopting healthy sleep habits is a vital step toward improving your overall wellness. By recognizing the role of sleep, establishing a consistent sleep routine, and addressing sleep disorders, when necessary, you can enhance your physical and mental well-being and enjoy a higher quality of life.

CHAPTER 8

Lifestyle and Habits

Your lifestyle and habits have a profound impact on your overall wellness.

8.1 Healthy Lifestyle Choices

Adopting healthy lifestyle choices is fundamental to achieving and maintaining overall wellness. Here are some key aspects of a healthy lifestyle:

Balanced Diet: Consume a balanced diet rich in fruits, vegetables, whole grains, lean proteins, and healthy fats. Pay attention to portion sizes and avoid excessive consumption of processed or sugary foods.

Regular Physical Activity: Engage in regular exercise and physical activity to maintain fitness, improve cardiovascular health, and manage weight.

Adequate Sleep: Prioritize sleep by establishing good sleep hygiene and ensuring you get enough restful sleep each night.

Stress Management: Practice stress-reduction techniques like mindfulness, meditation, and relaxation exercises to manage and mitigate stress.

Hydration: Stay properly hydrated by drinking an adequate amount of water throughout the day.

Moderation: Enjoy all things in moderation, including indulgent treats and occasional splurges. Avoid extreme diets or habits.

Limit Alcohol and Tobacco: If you consume alcohol, do so in moderation. Avoid smoking and limit exposure to secondhand smoke.

Regular Check-Ups: Schedule regular health check-ups with your healthcare provider to monitor your physical health and catch any potential issues early.

Mental Health Care: Prioritize your mental health by seeking therapy or counseling when needed. Mental well-being is as crucial as physical health.

Healthy Relationships: Cultivate positive and supportive relationships with friends and family. Healthy social connections are essential for emotional well-being.

Time Management: Organize your time effectively to reduce stress and maintain a work-life balance.

Hobbies and Interests: Engage in hobbies and interests that bring you joy and satisfaction. Pursuing your passions contributes to a fulfilling life.

8.2 Breaking Unhealthy Habits

Breaking unhealthy habits can be challenging but is essential for achieving wellness. Here are strategies to help you break unhealthy habits:

Identify the Habit: First, recognize the unhealthy habit you want to change. Be specific about what it is and why it's detrimental to your well-being.

Set Clear Goals: Establish clear and achievable goals for breaking the habit. Define what success looks like and set a timeline.

Replace with Positive Habits:
Replace the unhealthy habit with a healthier alternative. For example, replace smoking with chewing gum or taking short walks.

Seek Support: Share your goal with friends or family members who can offer encouragement and hold you accountable.

Understand Triggers: Identify the triggers or situations that lead to the unhealthy habit. Once you understand these triggers, you can develop strategies to avoid or manage them.

Use Positive Reinforcement: Reward yourself for making progress or achieving milestones in breaking the habit. Positive reinforcement can motivate you to continue.

Practice Mindfulness: Mindfulness techniques can help you become more aware of your habits and impulses. This self-awareness is key to breaking them.

Stay Patient: Breaking habits takes time, and setbacks are normal. Be patient with yourself and learn from your mistakes.

Professional Help: If needed, consider seeking professional help or counseling to address deeply ingrained habits or addictions.

8.3 Creating a Supportive Environment

Creating a supportive environment is essential for maintaining healthy lifestyle choices and breaking unhealthy habits. Here's how to foster a supportive environment:

Surround Yourself with Positivity: Spend time with people who support your wellness goals and encourage healthy habits.

Remove Temptations: Minimize exposure to environments or situations that trigger unhealthy habits. For example, if you're trying to quit smoking, avoid places where smoking is common.

Seek Accountability: Share your wellness goals with someone who can hold you accountable, such as a friend, family member, or coach.

Set Up Your Space: Organize your living and working spaces to support your wellness goals. This could include keeping healthy snacks on hand or creating a designated exercise area at home.

Educate Yourself: Stay informed about wellness topics and the latest research. Knowledge empowers you to make informed choices.

Build a Routine: Establish daily routines and rituals that prioritize wellness, such as morning stretching or a daily gratitude journal.

Social Support: Join clubs, groups, or online communities related to your wellness interests. Connecting with like-minded individuals can provide motivation and support.

Set Boundaries: Create boundaries that protect your well-being, such as limiting time spent on digital devices or saying no to commitments that cause stress.

Be Kind to Yourself: Practice self-compassion and avoid self-criticism. Understand that making positive changes takes time, and setbacks are part of the process.

A supportive environment is crucial for sustaining healthy lifestyle choices and breaking unhealthy habits. By surrounding yourself with positivity, removing obstacles, seeking accountability, and fostering a wellness-focused space, you can create an environment that empowers and motivates you to prioritize your well-being.

CHAPTER 9

Your Wellness Journey

Your wellness journey is a personal and ongoing process of self-improvement and well-being.

9.1 Tracking Your Progress

Tracking your progress is a vital aspect of your wellness journey. It helps you stay motivated, identify areas for improvement, and measure your achievements. Here's how to effectively track your progress:

Set Clear Goals: Begin by establishing clear and specific wellness goals. Whether it's improving fitness, losing weight, managing stress, or enhancing mental well-being, having well-defined objectives provides a roadmap for your journey.

Use Metrics: Whenever possible, use quantifiable metrics to measure your progress. For instance, track your weight, body measurements, exercise duration, or the number of days you practice stress-reduction techniques.

Keep a Journal: Maintain a wellness journal where you record your daily activities, thoughts, feelings, and behaviors related to your wellness goals. This journal can provide insights into patterns and triggers.

Use Technology: Consider using apps, wearables, or digital tools to track various aspects of your wellness journey. These tools can automate data collection and provide visual representations of your progress.

Regular Assessments: Schedule regular assessments or check-ins with yourself to evaluate how you're progressing toward your goals. These assessments can occur weekly, monthly, or at intervals that make sense for your objectives.

Celebrate Small Wins: Acknowledge and celebrate small victories along the way. Recognizing your achievements, no matter how minor they may seem, boosts motivation and reinforces positive behaviors.

Seek Feedback: Share your wellness journey with trusted friends, family members, or a wellness coach. Their feedback and support can be valuable in guiding your progress.

9.2 Adjusting Your Wellness Plan

Your wellness journey is not static; it's a dynamic process that may require adjustments over time. Here's how to make informed adjustments to your wellness plan:

Assess Your Results: Regularly review your progress and assess whether you're moving toward your goals. Reflect on what's working well and what might need improvement.

Be Flexible: Recognize that life is dynamic, and circumstances may change. Be open to adjusting your plan as needed to accommodate new challenges or opportunities.

Identify Barriers: If you encounter obstacles or barriers to your wellness goals, identify them. This might include time constraints, emotional challenges, or unexpected setbacks.

Reevaluate Goals: Periodically reevaluate your goals to ensure they remain relevant and achievable.

Adjust goals that no longer align with your priorities or interests.

Seek Expert Guidance: If you're unsure how to make necessary adjustments, consider seeking guidance from a wellness coach, nutritionist, personal trainer, or mental health professional. They can provide personalized advice and strategies.

Learn from Setbacks: Setbacks are a natural part of any wellness journey. Instead of viewing them as failures, see them as opportunities for learning and growth. Analyze what led to the setback and how you can prevent it in the future.

Stay Patient: Progress may not always be linear. There may be periods of rapid improvement followed by plateaus. Stay patient and persistent.

9.3 Celebrating Your Success

Celebrating your successes is an essential part of your wellness journey. It reinforces positive behaviors and provides motivation to continue striving for well-being. Here's how to celebrate your achievements:

Acknowledge Your Achievements: Take time to acknowledge and appreciate your accomplishments. Recognize the effort and dedication you've put into your wellness journey.

Reward Yourself: Consider rewarding yourself when you reach significant milestones or achieve specific goals. Rewards can be as simple as treating yourself to a favorite meal or indulging in a hobby you enjoy.

Share Your Success: Share your successes with friends and family who have supported you on your journey. Their encouragement and celebration can amplify your sense of achievement.

Set New Goals: After celebrating your successes, set new wellness goals to keep your journey evolving. Continuously striving for improvement can maintain your momentum.

Practice Gratitude: Cultivate gratitude for the progress you've made and the positive changes in your life. Gratitude can enhance your overall well-being.

Reflect on Your Journey: Reflect on how far you've come since the beginning of your wellness journey. Take pride in your accomplishments and the positive impact they've had on your life. wellness journey is a lifelong pursuit. By tracking your progress, making necessary adjustments, and celebrating your successes, you can navigate this journey with purpose and resilience, ultimately achieving and maintaining a higher level of well-being.

www.ingramcontent.com/pod-product-compliance
Lightning Source LLC
Chambersburg PA
CBHW060950260726
48661CB00005B/1821